How to Beat the Wheat:

Losing the Weight by Losing the Wheat in your Diet

This document is geared towards providing exact and reliable information in regards to the topic and issue covered. The publication is sold with the idea that the publisher is not required to render accounting, officially permitted, or otherwise, qualified services. If advice is necessary, legal or professional, a practiced individual in the profession should be ordered.

- From a Declaration of Principles which was accepted and approved equally by a Committee of the American Bar Association and a Committee of Publishers and Associations.

The information provided herein is stated to be truthful and consistent, in that any liability, in terms of inattention or otherwise, by any usage or abuse of any policies, processes, or directions contained within is the solitary and utter responsibility of the recipient reader. Under no circumstances will any

Introduction

I want to thank you and congratulate you for downloading the book, "How to Beat the Weight: Losing the Weight by Losing the Wheat in your Diet".

This book contains proven steps and strategies on how to lose the weight by simply dropping wheat from your diet. The first two chapters explain what it is in wheat that causes you to gain weight and how the concept of a wheat-free diet arose. The following two chapters outline the benefits of a wheat-free diet as well as the effects of consuming wheat. The final two chapters outline the challenging part of losing weight by losing wheat and also gives you guidance on how to remain focused. By the time you turn to the last page, you will have acquired essential knowledge to help you achieve your desired weight by losing wheat from your diet.

Thank you again for downloading this book, I hope you enjoy it!

Chapter 1

What does Wheat have?

Wheat contains gluten. Gluten is a component, also present in rye and barley, that is responsible for the elastic nature of the dough. Addition of gluten to low-protein food such as vegetarian meat alternatives increases the protein level in these foods. The addition of gluten to some food items like soy sauce and beer increases their shelf life and improves their flavor.

Gluten causes digestive upsets in individuals with gluten intolerance and intestinal damage in those with celiac disease. If you have celiac disease, the exclusion of gluten from your diet can help to alleviate the condition and have all the symptoms disappear if you take action at the early stages of the disease.

You might wonder how people discovered that removing the wheat from the diet causes weight loss. Initially, people did not remove wheat because they had celiac disease. Celiac disease refers to an autoimmune condition triggered by gluten from rye, barley and wheat. A good number of people also eliminated wheat from their diet because they were allergic to wheat.

Of those who eliminated wheat from their diet, about 40 percent recorded weight loss. Experts attributed weight loss to the exclusion of wheat and other grains from the diet. What is more, doctors are yet to diagnose celiac disease in most people, and if these people adopted a wheat-free diet, they would eventually lose weight.

Celebrities endorsed the trend of wheat-free diet, and it became popular as a weight loss diet. You will not have trouble adopting a wheat-free diet because it is simple to follow given that wheat-free products are now readily available in the market.

Chapter 2

Why Lose Wheat?

In your journey to lose weight by eliminating wheat you can enjoy the following benefits:

An average blood sugar level

Whenever you consume wheat, your body turns it into sugar rapidly. In fact, the conversion of grain into sugar begins the moment you bite into wheat made food—as digestion of wheat starts in the mouth. Wheat, therefore, belongs to a cluster of food with high glycemic index. Consumption of wheat immediately raises the level of insulin, a hormone that keeps blood sugar within the normal range in the body. It implies that whenever you take wheat, the level of insulin goes up, and the insulin converts excess sugar into fat for storage. Your body stores the fat under your body tissues and, as a result, you gain more weight. The sad thing is that the conversion of sugar to fat for storage causes a sugar crash making you feel hungry after a short while. You are then tempted to consume more food which will cause you to gain more weight as the cycle repeats itself.

A lean body

Carbohydrates are energy giving and essential for survival. However, you should be careful of the type of carbohydrates you consume. Some carbohydrates might do you more harm than good. Rather than eat a lot of wheat-containing food you should concentrate on eating more fruits and vegetables. You will simultaneously provide your body with carbohydrates and fiber that is essential for healthy bowel movement.

By including carbohydrates derived from gluten-free sources, you will achieve a lean, muscular and aesthetic body. Conversely, consumption of wheat and other grains that contain gluten will only make you gain more fat than muscle.

Decreased Risk of Diseases

If you do lose excess weight, you will develop a more desirable physique as well as improve your health. Excess weight is responsible for most of the lifestyle diseases such as hypertension, diabetes, and cardiovascular diseases. Wheat diet is responsible for causing high cholesterol that consequently causes the thickening of blood vessels. High blood pressure develops as your heart tries to pump blood through the narrowed vessels. Although wheat is not the only food type that causes dire health conditions, you should begin a healthy life by eliminating that which you know is harmful to your health—the gluten in wheat.

If you must eat foods that contain gluten, ensure that they undergo sprouting before converting them into edible products such as bread, cakes and cookies. By doing so, you will have eliminated some of the gluten and hence avoided problems caused by refined foods. The process of sprouting also increases the nutrients present in seeds while reducing the level of phytic acid, a component that hinders the absorption of minerals. Always go for products derived from sprouted grains when shopping for wheat or other grain products.

Chapter 3

Effects of Wheat

In the United States, 25 percent of people have Type 2 diabetes while 39 percent are pre-diabetic. In the past, these lifestyle diseases were not as common as they are today. The current health status of the modern generation has deteriorated over the years because in the 60's and especially the 80's, experts advised people to take more whole grains instead of fat and cholesterol-containing products.

The contemporary wheat is somewhat different from what our ancestors consumed approximately 1,000 years ago. The change in genetic composition of wheat is the source of the many wheat-diet related health problems. As aforementioned, wheat has a very high glycemic index, a glycemic index of 72 that is equal to or even more than that of table sugar with a glycemic index of 59.

If you have been looking for diets to enable you to lose weight, you have probably come across diets that substitute refined wheat flour for whole-wheat flour. Nevertheless, the truth is that you have to lose the wheat totally from your diet in order to achieve your weight loss objectives. Although promoters claim that the whole wheat is unrefined, the truth is that it is, but it contains bran to give it the brown color. The removal of the bran from wheat gives wheat flour a long shelf life.

Chapter 4

In the modern world with a whole range of wheat products, it is difficult to avoid wheat if you are undetermined to avoid it. You should make a decision to eat healthy to lose weight and achieve good health.

Consuming the following kind of food is recommended:

Quinoa

Quinoa is a grain that contains no gluten yet has a high content of protein. Experts recommend a serving of 8 grams. Quinoa also contains minerals such as magnesium and iron as well as fiber. Iron is necessary for processing of blood while magnesium is necessary for proper bone health and fiber aids in movement of the bowels.

Legumes

Legumes contain complex carbohydrate, vitamin B and Iron. These minerals are, usually, absent in most gluten free products making legumes a valuable food in wheat-free weight loss. Legumes include beans, peas and lentils. You can prepare legume dishes such as lentil soup and three-bean salad with ease.

Sweet potatoes

Sweet potatoes contain lots of antioxidants and fiber. Antioxidants ward off cancer while fiber aids in movement of bowels. Consumption of sweet potatoes thus helps to speed movement of materials in the gut. The faster materials move in the digestive system, the lesser the amount of absorbed material and hence no excess glucose to convert into fat for storage.

Popcorn

Although popcorn is a whole grain, it contains no gluten. By consuming popcorn, you provide your body with large quantities of antioxidants and fiber.

You should take popcorn to substitute wheat-made snacks. To make popcorn, use pop kernels or an air-popper in olive oil or canola oil on the top of your stovetop. You should then dust the stovetop with garlic, salt and any other natural seasoning of your choice.

Fruits and Vegetables

You should eat many green leafy vegetables. They contain a high content of fiber as well as vitamins.

Most fruits contain a high content of sugar. However, some have more sugar than others do. You should eat more of the low sugar fruit such as berries, oranges and apples. Avoid consumption of large quantities of bananas, mangoes, papayas and mangoes. The latter group of fruits contains a lot of sugar.

In addition to these food types, you should also eat the following: raw nuts, plant-derived oils (such as cocoa butter, olive and avocado), meat and eggs from grass-fed and free-range farm animals respectively. Besides these, you should eat full-fat cheese and ground flaxseeds.

You should eat limited quantities of soy including tofu, tempeh, natto and miso. Eat milk, butter, yogurt, and full-fat unsweetened cottage cheese in moderation. You should also eat moderate amounts of raw seeds, pickled vegetables, olives and avocados.

Chapter 5

Soy Sauce

From the name soy sauce, one would think that the sauce contains no wheat. Nevertheless, you will be shocked to find out that wheat is the main ingredient in the processing of soy sauce. If you must take soy sauce, look for tamari—a soy sauce traditionally made in Japan. The soy sauce by the brand name San-J is a gluten-free certified sauce. Another soy sauce that you may use is the Thai sauce. However, always ask the restaurant attendants whether it contains wheat as most restaurants in the United States use wheat to make Thai soy sauce.

Cream-Based Soups

Most people would never suspect that cream-based soups contained gluten. It is even difficult because the label mentions nothing about wheat. Most manufacturers use starch to achieve the texture of cream. The starch used comes from wheat hence large-scale manufacturers of canned soup use enormous quantity of wheat per annum.

In order to avoid consumption of wheat, be keen to read labels on products carefully. You should also consider purchasing costly soups instead of the cheap soups. The cheaper the soup is, the more likely it contains wheat.

Ice cream

It is unfortunate that most people expect ice cream to be a pure dairy product. However, in the contemporary world, you will be surprised to find out that it contains gluten as well. The familiar flavors such as "Key Lime Pie" and "Chocolate Chip Cookie Dough" contain gluten. Other brands are notorious of adding candies and cookies to their products to improve the flavor.

Some ice cream does not contain wheat as a product but as a thickener. Since most ice cream does contain gluten, you should be careful not to have your pure brand contaminated with wheat from other brands in your favorite ice cream shop. This contamination occurs as workers will use the same item to scoop different brands of ice cream.

It is prudent to identify a flavor that lacks gluten to ensure that you avoid eating ice cream that contains gluten. In addition, you should always ask the workers to get you a section from the back and to use a clean item when scooping the ice cream into your ice cream cup or container. You should also request that the worker use toppings from a new container as well.

Wheat-free products

Exclusion of wheat from your diet may enable you to lose weight. However, you can only achieve the results you desire if you exclude other gluten containing food from your diet. You should not concentrate on losing the wheat only but rather all products that have gluten. You will be subjecting yourself to more harm than good if you take a product that does not list wheat yet lists barley or rye among the ingredients.

Therefore, do not be fooled to believe those products that have the "wheat-free" label are the best for your weight loss adventure.

Beer

The standard beer contains gluten yet many people do not know. You will be doing zero work if you dutifully followed a wheat-free and gluten-free diet yet consumed beer. Beer factories use barley in the manufacture of beer; beer is, therefore, rich in gluten. However, some brands of beer are gluten free. If you must take beer, look for brands that have the "gluten-free" label on them. Although the beer does not have the taste of conventional beer, it is a good option if you want to lose weight.

Prescription Drugs

You will find that food labels indicate whether wheat is an ingredient or not. In contrast, the law does not require manufacturers of prescription drugs to provide a label indicating the ingredients of drugs. Pharmaceutical companies use wheat in the manufacturing of drugs as the filler. What is more, it is difficult to determine if a drug you are taking contains gluten. The contents of the drug may change and even the customer service representatives that could help you may not be aware of it.

To ensure that you are on track, let your pharmacist know that you cannot have gluten. In addition, always confirm that every single refill is similar to your last batch of gluten-free drugs.

Gourmet Meats

You will find gourmet meat in the form of sausages, pre-prepared ribs, and fish as well as chicken in most exclusive grocery stores. As delicious as the food may be, you are never sure of what the vendors use to prepare them. The stores get supplies of sauces and spices from other suppliers and tracking the ingredients used is tricky.

In the event that a worker assures you that an individual item does not have gluten, be careful because chances are that gluten from other sources such as bread crumbs could have contaminated it. Remember that the workers use the same meat counter when handling all types of meat.

Food from the Restaurant

You will realize that you must be careful of what you eat at the restaurant. By reading the menu, you might choose a particular food type while thinking that it is wheat-free. However, you should know that even the food that you think as wheat-free may have traces of gluten and could have contaminations by gluten from other foods in the same restaurant. For instance, hamburgers have breadcrumbs while marinades have soy sauce.

You will have to consult the server and sometimes the chef or manager in charge of the restaurant to be sure that your meal is wheat-free and gluten-free too. If you doubt that a particular food does not contain gluten, do not eat it!

Sharing meals with friends and Family

You should always remember that just because you should not eat gluten does not mean that other people around you are not going to eat it. It is very difficult to ensure that you do not take wheat or gluten when in the company of friends or family. It is even difficult to avoid taking gluten when hanging out with friends and family than it is in a restaurant.

For this reason, you should assist your family, or your friends to cook your food. The best thing is to prepare the food yourself but if you cannot, supervise a person who cooks, just to ensure that not even a drop of gluten finds its way into your food. Alternatively, carry food from your home if dining out with friends.

Other than the problem with food, friends and family may ask questions about your diet. Do not be tempted to taste their food to please them. In fact, if they challenge your decision to adopt a gluten/ wheat-free diet, affirm that you are okay with the choice of your diet as much as they are subtle with their food choices.

Chapter 6

Wheat free weight loss strategy

Losing wheat from your diet is not enough to make you lose weight to achieve the size that you desire. You will have to remain focused as well as combine the following strategies:

Get rid of processed gluten-free foods

Just because the food does not contain wheat or gluten does not guarantee you weight loss. Processed gluten-free products such as cookies, pizza, bread and snacks have more calories than most wheat products or gluten containing products. You must know the calories you take especially when you are looking forward to losing weight. You should always remember that absence of gluten from products does not mean that they do not have calories. If you do eat gluten-free products that are highly processed, you will only be adding more weight rather than losing it despite not taking wheat products.

Be keen on your total calorie uptake

For a successful weight loss with a wheat free diet, you need to watch your total calorie intake. Some people do go wheat-free but lose weight up to a certain point. In fact, experts claim that soon after excluding wheat and other gluten containing products from your diet, you will lose about 15 to 20 pounds. The initial weight loss occurs because lack of gluten decreases your urge to eat and your appetite in general. It implies that if you are to continue losing weight, you must be keen to calculate your calorie intake. You should make it a routine to avoid stagnation at a single point along your path to the desired weight.

Eat Paleo, low-carb and grain-free

Although the inclusion of a low carb diet is a controversial topic, experts agree that a low-carb diet applied alongside a wheat-free or gluten-free diet is effective for weight loss. The theory behind this recommendation is that all carbohydrates stimulate the production of insulin and make you feel hungry. You should take high-carb foods such as legumes and fruits in moderation and avoid gluten-free grain-based processed foods such as bread and cereals. You should also eliminate corn syrup as it contains a high content of fructose.

Focus on adopting a wheat-free and gluten-free diet

You should be capable of distinguishing between a gluten-free and wheat-free diet. You could think that you are on a gluten-free diet while you are not; gluten is present in food you would not suspect to have gluten. Experts suspect that even the smallest amount of gluten if taken on a regular basis, is capable of making you gaining weight. Although no research has confirmed this suspicion, you should avoid even minute traces of gluten in your diet. To achieve weight loss, you should not just eliminate wheat from your diet, but also any other food that contains gluten. Eliminating wheat only may be futile for weight loss: even if wheat is not present, the gluten in other products will make the insulin levels in your body to skyrocket.

Exercise

The best and healthiest way to lose weight is through a combination of the appropriate diet plus physical exercise. While dropping wheat and gluten from your diet may result into loss of a few pounds, exercise will make you reach your desired weight faster. It would be unfortunate to lose weight and remain with hanging skin where fat once existed. You should engage in physical activity in order to build more muscle and develop a lean body. Muscle enables the body to burn even more fat thus ensuring that you lose weight and achieve fitness.

Do's and Don'ts for a successful wheat-free weight loss

Eat eight or more servings of vegetables every day.

Eat four servings of berries or fresh fruits every day.

Eat 30 grams of protein after every 2-3 hours.

Take eight glasses of water or green tea every day

Do not eat processed grains such as muffins, bread and donuts.

Do not eat whole-wheat, barley and whole-rye.

Do not eat sugar-based products such as sweets, candy and soda.

Sleep 7 to 9 hours every night.

Avoid stress.

Enjoy every step of the transformation—it will amaze you how happy you can be!

Conclusion

Thank you again for downloading this book!

I hope this book was able to help you know how to lose excess weight by eliminating wheat from your diet.

The next step is to follow each of the steps outlined here to achieve a healthy weight and rebuild your esteem.

Finally, if you enjoyed this book, then I'd like to ask you for a favor, would you be kind enough to leave a review for this book on Amazon? It'd be greatly appreciated!